The
Vitamins
and
Minerals
Book

Essential Nutrients for Good Health

Janet DiBiase

Contents

Introduction

The human body, a marvel of biological engineering, is composed of a complex interplay of elements, each contributing to its intricate structure and function. Surprisingly, a mere six elements—oxygen, carbon, hydrogen, nitrogen, calcium, and phosphorus—account for approximately 99% of our body mass. These fundamental elements form the very scaffolding of our being, from the oxygen we breathe to the calcium that fortifies our bones. They are integral to the construction of proteins, carbohydrates, lipids, and nucleic acids, the essential biomolecules that drive every process within us. Oxygen, for instance, is vital for cellular respiration, the process that converts food into energy. Carbon forms the backbone of all organic molecules, while hydrogen plays a crucial role in maintaining pH balance and transporting nutrients. Nitrogen is a key component of amino acids, the building blocks of proteins, and calcium provides structural integrity to our skeletal system. Phosphorus, working in concert with calcium, is essential for bone health and also plays a critical role in energy metabolism.

Beyond these foundational six, another five elements—potassium, sulfur, sodium, chlorine, and magnesium—contribute a further 0.85% of our body mass. While present in smaller quantities, their roles are no less critical. Potassium and sodium, for example, work together to regulate fluid balance, nerve impulses, and muscle contractions. Sulfur is a component of certain amino acids and vitamins, contributing to protein structure and function. Chlorine is crucial for maintaining proper fluid balance and stomach acid production. Magnesium plays a vital role in over 300 biochemical reactions in the body, including protein synthesis, muscle and nerve function, blood glucose control, and blood pressure regulation. Together, these elements orchestrate a symphony of biological processes that keep us functioning optimally.

The remaining fraction, less than 0.01% of our body mass, comprises a collection of elements known as trace minerals. Though present in minute quantities, these trace elements are indispensable for optimal health. This seemingly insignificant percentage belies the profound impact these micronutrients have on our well-being. These essential elements act as catalysts and co-factors in a vast array of biochemical reactions, influencing everything from energy production and immune function to hormone regulation and antioxidant defense. Understanding the roles of both vitamins and minerals is crucial for maintaining vibrant health and preventing disease.

Vitamins, organic compounds obtained primarily through our diet, are essential for normal growth and development. They are categorized into two groups based on their solubility: water-soluble and fat-soluble. Water-soluble vitamins, including vitamin C and the B vitamins, are not stored in the body to a significant degree and therefore require regular replenishment through our diet. These vitamins play diverse roles, from supporting the immune system (Vitamin C) to facilitating energy production and maintaining nerve health (B Vitamins). Fat-soluble vitamins, such as vitamins A, D, E, and K, are stored in the body's fatty tissues and liver. Vitamin A is crucial for vision, immune function, and cell growth. Vitamin D plays a key role in calcium absorption and bone health. Vitamin E acts as an antioxidant, protecting cells from damage. Vitamin K is essential for blood clotting.

Minerals, unlike vitamins, are inorganic substances. They too are categorized by the amount required by the body: macrominerals and trace minerals. Macrominerals, needed in larger amounts, include calcium, phosphorus, magnesium, sodium, potassium, chloride, and sulfur. These minerals perform a diverse range of functions, from building strong bones and teeth (calcium and phosphorus) to regulating fluid balance (sodium and potassium) and supporting muscle function (magnesium). Trace minerals, required in much smaller amounts, include iron, zinc, copper, manganese, selenium, iodine, fluoride, molybdenum, chromium, and cobalt. Despite their minute requirements, they are essential for a variety of bodily processes. Iron, for example, is crucial for transporting oxygen throughout the body. Zinc supports immune function and wound healing. Iodine is essential for thyroid hormone production, which regulates metabolism. Other trace minerals, like chromium, molybdenum, and cobalt, play important roles in enzyme function and various metabolic processes. While less common, other elements like boron, silicon, arsenic, and lithium are also considered essential trace elements, although their precise roles in human health are still being investigated.

A balanced diet rich in fruits, vegetables, whole grains, lean proteins, and dairy products is the cornerstone of obtaining adequate vitamins and minerals. However, individual needs vary, and some individuals may benefit from supplementation due to specific deficiencies, dietary restrictions, or health conditions. This book will delve into the fascinating world of vitamins and minerals, exploring their individual functions, recommended intakes, potential deficiency symptoms, and food sources. Understanding the intricate roles these micronutrients play empowers us to make informed choices about our nutrition and optimize our health and well-being.

The Essential Elements: Foundations of Human Life

The human body, a complex and dynamic system, relies on a delicate balance of elements for its structure and function. While numerous elements are present, six stand out as essential: oxygen, carbon, hydrogen, nitrogen, calcium, and phosphorus. These elements, comprising nearly 99% of our body mass, form the very foundation of our being, participating in countless biological processes essential for life.

Oxygen (O): The Breath of Life

Oxygen is arguably the most critical element for human survival. It plays a central role in cellular respiration, the process by which cells convert glucose and other nutrients into adenosine triphosphate (ATP), the body's primary energy currency. This energy fuels every physiological process, from muscle contraction and nerve impulse transmission to cell division and growth. Oxygen is also a key component of water, which constitutes approximately 60% of the human body and serves as a solvent for vital nutrients, a transport medium for hormones and waste products, and a regulator of body temperature. Furthermore, oxygen is a component of numerous other essential molecules, including proteins, carbohydrates, and lipids. Without a constant supply of oxygen, cellular function rapidly deteriorates, leading to organ damage and ultimately, death.

Carbon (C): The Backbone of Life's Molecules

Carbon is unique in its ability to form long chains and complex structures, making it the fundamental building block of all organic molecules. These molecules, including proteins, carbohydrates, lipids, and nucleic acids (DNA and RNA), are essential for life. Proteins, composed of amino acids linked together by carbon atoms, serve as structural components of cells, enzymes that catalyze biochemical reactions, and signaling molecules that regulate cellular processes. Carbohydrates, another class of carbon-based molecules, provide a readily available source of energy. Lipids, including fats and oils, store energy, form cell membranes, and act as signaling molecules. Nucleic acids, DNA and RNA, carry the genetic information that dictates the synthesis of proteins and governs heredity.

Hydrogen (H): A Versatile Partner in Life's Chemistry

Hydrogen, the most abundant element in the universe, plays a crucial role in human biology. Like oxygen, it is a component of water, the life-sustaining solvent that permeates every cell and tissue. Hydrogen ions (H+) are essential for maintaining the body's delicate acid-base balance, or pH, which is critical for enzyme activity and overall cellular function. Hydrogen also participates in numerous biochemical reactions, including energy production and the synthesis of essential molecules.

Furthermore, hydrogen bonds, weak attractions between hydrogen atoms and other electronegative atoms like oxygen and nitrogen, are crucial for maintaining the three-dimensional structure of proteins and nucleic acids, which is essential for their function.

Nitrogen (N): Essential for Proteins and Genetic Information

Nitrogen is a vital component of amino acids, the building blocks of proteins. Proteins, as previously mentioned, are involved in virtually every aspect of cellular function, from structural support and enzymatic catalysis to cell signaling and immune defense. Nitrogen is also a key component of nucleic acids, DNA and RNA, the molecules that store and transmit genetic information. DNA carries the blueprint for all the proteins synthesized in the body, while RNA plays a crucial role in protein synthesis and gene regulation. Without sufficient nitrogen, the body cannot synthesize the proteins and nucleic acids necessary for growth, repair, and maintenance of tissues.

Calcium (Ca): The Guardian of Bones and More

Calcium is the most abundant mineral in the human body, with approximately 99% residing in bones and teeth, providing structural integrity and strength. However, calcium also plays crucial roles outside the skeletal system. It is essential for muscle contraction, nerve impulse transmission, blood clotting, and the regulation of various enzymes. Calcium ions ($Ca2+$) act as signaling molecules, triggering cellular responses involved in hormone secretion, muscle contraction, and nerve function. Maintaining proper calcium balance is crucial for overall health, and deficiencies can lead to osteoporosis, muscle cramps, and nerve dysfunction.

Phosphorus (P): Partnering with Calcium and Powering Cells

Phosphorus, the second most abundant mineral in the body, works closely with calcium to build and maintain strong bones and teeth. However, phosphorus also plays crucial roles in energy metabolism, cell signaling, and the structure of cell membranes. It is a key component of ATP, the primary energy currency of cells. Phosphorus is also a component of phospholipids, the molecules that form the structural framework of cell membranes. Furthermore, phosphorus is a component of DNA and RNA, the carriers of genetic information. Maintaining adequate phosphorus levels is essential for energy production, cellular function, and overall health.

These six essential elements – oxygen, carbon, hydrogen, nitrogen, calcium, and phosphorus – form the fundamental building blocks of the human body and are essential for life. Their intricate interplay in countless biochemical reactions and structural components underscores the remarkable complexity and efficiency of human biology.

Essential Nutrients: Fueling a Healthy Life

The human body is a complex machine that requires a diverse array of nutrients to function optimally. These essential nutrients, obtained through the food we consume, play vital roles in everything from energy production and cell repair to immune function and hormone regulation. Understanding the roles and sources of these nutrients empowers us to make informed dietary choices that support our health and well-being.

Proteins: The Building Blocks of Life

Proteins are essential for building and repairing tissues, including muscles, organs, skin, and hair. They are composed of amino acids, the "building blocks" of protein. The body can synthesize some amino acids, but others, known as essential amino acids, must be obtained through the diet. Proteins also play crucial roles in:

Enzyme Production: Enzymes, biological catalysts that speed up chemical reactions, are primarily made of protein.
Hormone Synthesis: Many hormones, chemical messengers that regulate bodily functions, are protein-based.
Antibody Formation: Antibodies, crucial components of the immune system, are proteins that help defend the body against infection.
Energy Production: While carbohydrates and fats are the primary energy sources, protein can be used for energy when these sources are depleted.

Dietary Sources: Meat, poultry, fish, eggs, dairy products, beans, lentils, nuts, seeds, and soy products are excellent sources of protein.

Fats: Essential for Energy, Protection, and Hormone Production

Fats, often demonized, are crucial for numerous bodily functions. They provide a concentrated source of energy, storing more than twice the calories per gram compared to carbohydrates or proteins. Fats also:
Insulate and Protect Organs: A layer of fat surrounds vital organs, cushioning them from impact and helping regulate body temperature.
Aid in Fat-Soluble Vitamin Absorption: Vitamins A, D, E, and K are fat-soluble, meaning they require fat for proper absorption.
Contribute to Hormone Production: Certain hormones, including sex hormones, are synthesized from fats.

Form Cell Membranes: Fats are essential components of cell membranes, maintaining their structure and function.

Types of Fats:
Unsaturated Fats (Healthy Fats): Found in avocados, nuts, seeds, olive oil, and fatty fish. These fats are liquid at room temperature and can help lower cholesterol levels and reduce the risk of heart disease.
Saturated Fats: Found in red meat, poultry skin, dairy products, and coconut oil. These fats are solid at room temperature and should be consumed in moderation.
Trans Fats (Unhealthy Fats): Found in processed foods, fried foods, and some baked goods. These fats should be avoided as they raise LDL ("bad") cholesterol and increase the risk of heart disease.

Carbohydrates: The Body's Primary Fuel Source

Carbohydrates are the body's preferred source of energy. They are broken down into glucose, which cells use for fuel.
Types of Carbohydrates:
Sugars (Simple Carbohydrates): Found naturally in fruits, vegetables, milk, and honey. Also found in processed foods like candy, sugary drinks, and desserts. While naturally occurring sugars are acceptable in moderation, added sugars should be limited.
Starches (Complex Carbohydrates): Found in starchy vegetables (potatoes, corn), grains (rice, wheat, oats), and legumes (beans, lentils). Complex carbohydrates provide sustained energy and are generally healthier than simple sugars.
Fiber (Complex Carbohydrate): Indigestible by humans, fiber plays a crucial role in digestive health, promoting regularity, and preventing constipation. It also helps regulate blood sugar levels and can contribute to feelings of fullness, aiding in weight management. Excellent sources of fiber include whole grains, fruits, vegetables, legumes, nuts, and seeds.

Vitamins: Essential Micronutrients for Diverse Functions

Vitamins are organic compounds required in small amounts for a wide range of bodily functions. They are classified as either fat-soluble (A, D, E, and K) or water-soluble (C and B vitamins).
Fat-Soluble Vitamins: Stored in the body's fatty tissues and liver.
Water-Soluble Vitamins: Not stored in large amounts and need to be replenished regularly through the diet.
Vitamins play crucial roles in immune function, vision, bone health, energy production, and numerous other processes.

Minerals: Inorganic Essentials for Structure and Function
Minerals are inorganic substances essential for various bodily functions. They are classified as macrominerals (needed in larger amounts) and trace minerals (needed in smaller amounts).
Macrominerals: Include calcium, phosphorus, magnesium, sodium, potassium, chloride, and sulfur.
Trace Minerals: Include iron, zinc, copper, manganese, selenium, iodine, fluoride, chromium, and molybdenum.

Minerals contribute to bone health, nerve function, muscle contraction, fluid balance, oxygen transport, and enzyme activity.

Water: The Elixir of Life
Water is essential for all life processes. It makes up a significant portion of body weight and is involved in:

Digestion and Absorption: Water helps break down food and absorb nutrients.
Transportation of Nutrients: Water carries nutrients throughout the body.
Waste Removal: Water flushes out waste products through urine and sweat.
Temperature Regulation: Water helps maintain body temperature through sweating.
Lubrication of Joints: Water acts as a lubricant for joints and cushions organs.

Essential Fatty Acids: Crucial for Brain Health and Inflammation Control
Essential fatty acids, including omega-3 and omega-6 fatty acids, are necessary fats that the body cannot produce on its own. They must be obtained through the diet. These fatty acids play crucial roles in:
Brain Function: Essential for cognitive development and function.
Inflammation Control: Omega-3 fatty acids have anti-inflammatory properties.
Cell Growth: Essential for cell membrane structure and function.

Dietary Sources: Fatty fish (salmon, tuna, mackerel), flaxseed oil, chia seeds, and walnuts are good sources of omega-3 fatty acids. Vegetable oils (corn oil, soybean oil) and nuts are sources of omega-6 fatty acids.

By consuming a balanced diet that includes a variety of nutrient-rich foods, we can ensure we are providing our bodies with the essential nutrients they need to thrive. This includes focusing on whole, unprocessed foods like fruits, vegetables, whole grains, lean proteins, and healthy fats. While supplements can be helpful in certain situations, it's always best to obtain nutrients from food whenever possible.

The Benefits of Vitamins and Minerals

Vitamins and minerals, though needed only in small amounts, are essential micronutrients that play a pivotal role in maintaining overall health and well-being. These vital nutrients act as catalysts and co-factors in countless biochemical reactions, influencing a vast array of physiological processes. From bolstering the immune system and supporting growth and development to protecting against chronic diseases and enhancing cognitive function, the benefits of vitamins and minerals are profound and far-reaching.

Bolstering the Immune System: The Body's Defense Force

A robust immune system is crucial for defending the body against invading pathogens, such as bacteria, viruses, and fungi. Several vitamins and minerals play critical roles in supporting immune function:

Vitamin C: A potent antioxidant, vitamin C enhances the function of various immune cells, including white blood cells that engulf and destroy pathogens.
Vitamin D: Plays a crucial role in immune regulation, modulating both innate and adaptive immune responses.
Zinc: Essential for the development and function of immune cells. Zinc deficiency can impair immune function and increase susceptibility to infections.
Selenium: An essential component of selenoproteins, which have antioxidant and anti-inflammatory properties that support immune function.

Supporting Growth and Development: Building a Healthy Foundation

Vitamins and minerals are essential for proper growth and development throughout the lifespan, particularly during childhood and adolescence. These nutrients are crucial for:

Bone and Teeth Formation: Calcium, phosphorus, vitamin D, and magnesium are essential for building strong bones and teeth.
Muscle Development: Protein, magnesium, and potassium are crucial for muscle growth and function.

Cognitive Development: Iron, zinc, iodine, and various B vitamins are essential for brain development and cognitive function.

Enhancing Energy Production: Fueling the Body's Engine

Energy production, the process by which the body converts food into usable energy, relies on several key vitamins and minerals:

B Vitamins: B vitamins, including thiamine (B1), riboflavin (B2), niacin (B3), pantothenic acid (B5), pyridoxine (B6), and cobalamin (B12), play essential roles in various metabolic pathways involved in energy production.
Iron: Essential for the formation of hemoglobin, the protein in red blood cells that carries oxygen throughout the body. Adequate oxygen supply is crucial for efficient energy production.
Magnesium: Involved in over 300 biochemical reactions in the body, including those involved in energy metabolism.

Promoting Healthy Skin, Hair, and Nails: Reflecting Inner Health

The health of our skin, hair, and nails often reflects our overall nutritional status. Several vitamins and minerals contribute to their health and vitality:

Vitamin A: Essential for cell growth and differentiation, contributing to healthy skin and mucous membranes.
Vitamin E: A potent antioxidant that protects skin cells from damage caused by free radicals.
Biotin: Plays a role in the production of keratin, a key protein that makes up hair, skin, and nails.
Zinc: Essential for cell growth and repair, contributing to healthy skin, hair, and nail growth.

Supporting Brain Function: Sharpening the Mind

The brain, a complex and energy-demanding organ, relies on a variety of nutrients for optimal function. Several vitamins and minerals play crucial roles in supporting cognitive health:
Omega-3 Fatty Acids: Essential components of brain cell membranes, supporting cognitive function and reducing the risk of age-related cognitive decline.

B Vitamins: Essential for nerve function and neurotransmitter synthesis, impacting mood, memory, and cognitive performance.
Vitamin E: An antioxidant that protects brain cells from oxidative damage.
Magnesium: Plays a role in nerve transmission and synaptic plasticity, supporting learning and memory.

Maintaining Healthy Vision: Protecting the Windows to the World

Vitamins and minerals are essential for maintaining good vision and protecting against age-related eye diseases:

Vitamin A: Crucial for the formation of rhodopsin, a light-sensitive pigment in the retina essential for vision in low light.
Vitamin C: An antioxidant that protects eye tissues from oxidative damage.
Vitamin E: May help protect against age-related macular degeneration and cataracts.
Zinc and Selenium: Antioxidants that protect eye cells from damage.

Supporting Heart Health: Maintaining a Strong Cardiovascular System

A healthy heart is essential for overall health and longevity. Several vitamins and minerals contribute to cardiovascular health:

Vitamin D: May play a role in regulating blood pressure and reducing inflammation.
Vitamin K: Essential for blood clotting, preventing excessive bleeding.
Magnesium: Helps regulate blood pressure and muscle function, including heart muscle.
Potassium: Helps regulate blood pressure and fluid balance.

Enhancing Bone Health: Building a Strong Framework

Strong bones are essential for mobility, support, and protection of internal organs. Several nutrients are crucial for bone health:

Calcium: The most abundant mineral in the body, providing structural integrity to bones and teeth.
Vitamin D: Essential for calcium absorption and bone mineralization.
Magnesium and Phosphorus: Also contribute to bone structure and strength.

Supporting a Healthy Pregnancy: Nourishing Mother and Baby

Adequate intake of vitamins and minerals is especially crucial during pregnancy for the health of both the mother and the developing fetus:

Folic Acid: Essential for preventing neural tube defects in the developing fetus.
Iron: Needed to support the increased blood volume during pregnancy and prevent anemia.
Calcium and Vitamin D: Crucial for fetal bone development.

Protecting Against Oxidative Stress: Combating Cellular Damage

Oxidative stress, caused by an imbalance between free radicals and antioxidants, can damage cells and contribute to chronic diseases. Many vitamins and minerals act as antioxidants, protecting against this damage:

Vitamins C and E: Potent antioxidants that neutralize free radicals.
Selenium and Zinc: Essential components of antioxidant enzymes.

By consuming a balanced diet rich in fruits, vegetables, whole grains, lean proteins, and healthy fats, we can ensure adequate intake of these essential vitamins and minerals. In some cases, supplementation may be necessary to address specific deficiencies or health concerns.

Vitamins

Vitamins are organic compounds that are essential for the normal functioning of the body. They are required in small amounts and cannot be produced by the body in sufficient quantities, so they must be obtained from the diet.

Vitamins play crucial roles in various physiological processes, including metabolism, growth, development, and maintaining overall health. They act as coenzymes or cofactors in enzymatic reactions, facilitating the conversion of food into energy and supporting numerous biochemical reactions in the body.

There are two types of vitamins:

Water-soluble Vitamins: These include vitamins C and the B-complex vitamins (B1, B2, B3, B5, B6, B7, B9, and B12). They are soluble in water and are not stored in the body to a significant extent. Water-soluble vitamins are easily absorbed into the bloodstream and any excess is excreted through urine.

Fat-soluble Vitamins: These include vitamins A, D, E, and K. They are soluble in fats and oils and are stored in the body's fat tissues.

Fat-soluble vitamins are absorbed along with dietary fats and are best absorbed when consumed with fat-containing foods.

Vitamin A

Vitamin A is a fat-soluble vitamin that is essential for various bodily functions. It plays a crucial role in maintaining healthy vision, promoting growth and development, supporting the immune system, and maintaining the health of the skin and mucous membranes.

There are two forms of vitamin A: retinoids and carotenoids. Both forms of vitamin A are important for maintaining healthy vision, immune function, and skin health.

Retinoids: Retinol, retinal, and retinoic acid, are found in animal sources like liver, fish, and dairy products. Retinoids are the active form of vitamin A that can be directly used by the body.

Carotenoids: Beta-carotene, are a provitamin form of vitamin A found in plant-based foods like carrots, sweet potatoes, and spinach. The body converts carotenoids into retinoids, which are then utilized for various functions in the body.

Vitamin A is important for maintaining good vision, especially in low-light conditions. It is a component of rhodopsin, a protein in the retina that helps with night vision. Deficiency of vitamin A can lead to night blindness and other vision problems.

Vitamin A also plays a role in promoting growth and development, particularly in children. It is necessary for the proper development of bones, teeth, and soft tissues.

It also supports the immune system by helping to maintain the integrity of the skin and mucous membranes, which act as barriers against pathogens.

Vitamin A is involved in the production and maintenance of healthy skin cells. It helps to regulate the production of sebum, an oily substance that moisturizes the skin and prevents dryness. Vitamin A deficiency can lead to dry, rough, and flaky skin.

While vitamin A is important for overall health, it is essential to consume it in appropriate amounts. Excessive intake of vitamin A, particularly from supplements, can be toxic and lead to symptoms such as nausea, dizziness, and even liver damage. It is recommended to obtain vitamin A from a balanced diet rather than relying solely on supplements. The daily recommended intake of vitamin A for children is 300-600 micrograms (mcg) depending on age, and for adults, it is 700-900 mcg depending on gender and age.

Recommended Dietary Allowance (RDA): For men ages 19 and older is 900 mcg (3,00 IU) daily, and for women ages 19 and older is 700 mcg (2,333 IU) daily.

Foods sources of Vitamin A:

Beef liver: Beef liver is one of the richest sources of vitamin A. A 3-ounce serving of beef liver can provide more than 600% of the daily recommended intake of vitamin A.

Eggs: Eggs contain a moderate amount of vitamin A, primarily in the yolk. One large egg typically contains approximately 75-80 micrograms (mcg) of Vitamin A or about 6% of the daily recommended intake of vitamin A.

Shrimp: Shrimp is a good source of vitamin A. A 3-ounce serving of shrimp can provide about 10% of the daily recommended intake of vitamin A and 100 grams of cooked shrimp typically contain about 590 micrograms (mcg) of Vitamin A.

Fish: Certain types of fish, such as salmon and mackerel, contain small amounts of vitamin A. However, the vitamin A content in fish is generally lower compared to other sources.

Fortified milk: Many brands of milk are fortified with vitamin A. One cup of fortified milk can provide about 10% of the daily recommended intake of vitamin A.

Sweet potatoes: Sweet potatoes are an excellent source of vitamin A. One medium-sized sweet potato can provide more than 400% of the daily recommended intake of vitamin A.

Carrots: Carrots are well-known for their high vitamin A content. One medium-sized carrot can provide about 200% of the daily recommended intake of vitamin A.

Pumpkins: Pumpkins are also rich in vitamin A. One cup of cooked pumpkin can provide about 200% of the daily recommended intake of vitamin A.

Spinach: Spinach is a good source of vitamin A. One cup of cooked spinach can provide about 100% of the daily recommended intake of vitamin A.

Mangoes: Mangoes contain a moderate amount of vitamin A. One medium-sized mango can provide about 20% of the daily recommended intake of vitamin A.

The B-Vitamin Complex

The B-vitamin complex consists of eight different vitamins: thiamine (B1), riboflavin (B2), niacin (B3), pantothenic acid (B5), pyridoxine (B6), biotin (B7), folate (B9), and cobalamin (B12). These vitamins play important roles in various metabolic processes in the body.

Vitamin B1 (Thiamine)

Vitamin B1, also known as thiamine, is a water-soluble vitamin that is essential for the proper functioning of the body. It plays a crucial role in converting food into energy and is involved in various metabolic processes.

Thiamine is primarily involved in the metabolism of carbohydrates. It helps to convert glucose into energy that the body can use. It is an important coenzyme in the production of ATP (adenosine triphosphate), which is the main energy currency of the body.

Thiamine also plays a role in the proper functioning of the nervous system. It is involved in the synthesis of neurotransmitters, which are chemical messengers that transmit signals between nerve cells. Thiamine deficiency can lead to neurological symptoms such as confusion, memory problems, and muscle weakness.

Thiamine is important for maintaining a healthy cardiovascular system. It helps in the production of red blood cells and supports the proper functioning of the heart. Thiamine deficiency can lead to a condition called beriberi, which is characterized by cardiovascular problems such as an enlarged heart and heart failure.

It is important to consume a balanced diet to ensure an adequate intake of thiamine. However, certain factors such as alcoholism, malabsorption disorders, and certain medical conditions can increase the risk of thiamine deficiency.

Foods sources of Vitamin B1:
Whole grains: Whole grains, such as brown rice, whole wheat bread, oatmeal, and quinoa, are excellent sources of vitamin B1. They provide a significant amount of thiamine and are also rich in other nutrients and fiber.
Legumes: Legumes, including lentils, black beans, chickpeas, and kidney beans, are high in thiamine. They are not only a good source of vitamin B1 but also provide protein, fiber, and other essential nutrients.

Nuts and seeds: Nuts and seeds, such as sunflower seeds, flaxseeds, peanuts, and pistachios, contain thiamine. They are also packed with healthy fats, protein, and other vitamins and minerals.

Pork: Pork is one of the best animal sources of thiamine. It provides a significant amount of vitamin B1, along with other nutrients like protein and iron. However, it is important to choose lean cuts of pork to minimize saturated fat intake.

Fish: Certain types of fish, such as tuna, trout, and salmon, contain thiamine. Fish is also a good source of omega-3 fatty acids, which have numerous health benefits.

Fortified cereals: Some breakfast cereals are fortified with thiamine and other B vitamins. Check the nutrition labels to find cereals that provide a good amount of vitamin B1.

Yeast extract: Yeast extract, such as nutritional yeast, is a popular ingredient in vegan and vegetarian diets. It is a good source of thiamine and can be used as a flavoring or nutritional supplement.

Pork liver: Pork liver is another animal source of thiamine. It is rich in vitamin B1, as well as other nutrients like iron and vitamin A. However, it is important to consume liver in moderation due to its high cholesterol content.

Oranges: Oranges and other citrus fruits contain a small amount of thiamine. While they are not a significant source of vitamin B1, they are still a healthy addition to a balanced diet due to their high vitamin C content.

Recommended Dietary Allowance (RDA): For men ages 19 and older is 1.2 mg daily, and for women ages 19 and older is 1.2 mg daily.

Vitamin B2 (Riboflavin)

Vitamin B2, also known as riboflavin, is a water-soluble vitamin that is essential for various bodily functions. It plays a crucial role in energy production, growth, and development, as well as maintaining the health of the skin, eyes, and nervous system.

Riboflavin is involved in the metabolism of carbohydrates, fats, and proteins. It helps convert these macronutrients into energy that the body can use. Riboflavin is a component of two important coenzymes, flavin adenine dinucleotide (FAD) and flavin mononucleotide (FMN), which are involved in numerous enzymatic reactions in the body. In addition to its role in energy production, riboflavin is important for the growth and development of tissues. It is necessary for the synthesis of DNA, RNA, and other important molecules involved in cell division and growth. Riboflavin also plays a role in the production of red blood cells and the maintenance of healthy skin, hair, and nails. Riboflavin is also essential for maintaining the health of the eyes and the nervous system. It is involved in the production of glutathione, an important antioxidant that helps protect the eyes from oxidative damage. Riboflavin deficiency can lead to eye problems such as sensitivity to light and blurred vision.

Riboflavin is also involved in the production of neurotransmitters, which are chemical messengers that transmit signals between nerve cells. It is not stored in the body, so it needs to be consumed regularly through the diet. However, riboflavin deficiency is rare in developed countries, as it is found in a wide variety of foods.
Riboflavin deficiency can lead to a condition called ariboflavinosis, which is characterized by symptoms such as sore throat, swollen and cracked lips, and inflamed tongue. Riboflavin deficiency can be treated with riboflavin supplements or by increasing the intake of riboflavin-rich foods.
Riboflavin is a water-soluble vitamin, which means it is not stored in the body and needs to be replenished regularly through diet.

Foods sources of Vitamin B2:
Dairy products: Milk, yogurt, and cheese are excellent sources of riboflavin. They provide a significant amount of vitamin B2, along with other nutrients like calcium and protein.
Eggs: Eggs are a good source of riboflavin. One large egg provides about 15% of the daily recommended intake of vitamin B2.
Lean meats: Lean meats, such as chicken breast and turkey, contain riboflavin. They are also rich in protein and other essential nutrients.
Organ meats: Organ meats, such as liver and kidneys, are particularly high in riboflavin. However, they should be consumed in moderation due to their high cholesterol content.
Fish: Certain types of fish, such as salmon and trout, contain riboflavin. Fish is also a good source of omega-3 fatty acids, which have numerous health benefits.
Fortified cereals: Some breakfast cereals are fortified with riboflavin and other B vitamins. Check the nutrition labels to find cereals that provide a good amount of vitamin B2.
Mushrooms: Mushrooms, such as crimini and portobello mushrooms, contain riboflavin. They are also low in calories and a good source of fiber.
Spinach: Spinach and other leafy green vegetables contain riboflavin. They are also packed with other vitamins, minerals, and antioxidants.
Almonds: Almonds and other nuts are a good source of riboflavin. They are also rich in healthy fats, protein, and other nutrients.
Soybeans: Soybeans and soy products, such as tofu and tempeh, contain riboflavin. They are also a good source of plant-based protein.

Vitamin B3 (Niacin)

Vitamin B3, also known as niacin, is a water-soluble vitamin that is essential for various bodily functions. It plays a crucial role in energy production, DNA repair, and the maintenance of healthy skin, nerves, and digestion.

Niacin is involved in the metabolism of carbohydrates, fats, and proteins. It helps convert these macronutrients into energy that the body can use.

Niacin is a component of two important coenzymes, nicotinamide adenine dinucleotide (NAD) and nicotinamide adenine dinucleotide phosphate (NADP), which are involved in numerous enzymatic reactions in the body. In addition to its role in energy production, niacin is important for the synthesis and repair of DNA. It is involved in the production of genetic material and helps maintain the integrity of the DNA molecule. It also plays a role in the production of certain hormones and neurotransmitters. It is essential for maintaining the health of the skin, nerves, and digestion. It helps maintain the integrity of the skin and mucous membranes, which act as barriers against pathogens.

Niacin is also involved in the production of myelin, a protective covering around nerve cells that helps with the transmission of nerve signals. Additionally, niacin plays a role in the production of digestive enzymes that help break down food and absorb nutrients.

It can be synthesized in the body from the amino acid tryptophan, which is found in protein-rich foods. However, niacin deficiency can occur in individuals who have a poor diet or certain medical conditions that affect nutrient absorption.

Niacin deficiency can lead to a condition called pellagra, which is characterized by symptoms such as dermatitis (skin inflammation), diarrhea, dementia, and even death if left untreated.

Recommended Dietary Allowance (RDA): For men ages 19 and older is 16 mg daily, for women ages 19 and older is 14 mg daily, for pregnant women is 18 mg daily and for lactating women is 17 mg daily.

Foods sources of Vitamin B3:

Chicken breast: 100g provides about 14.9 mg of niacin.

Tuna: 100g contains approximately 11.3 mg of niacin.

Salmon: 100g offers around 8.6 mg of niacin.

Pork chops: 100g provides about 4.5 mg of niacin.

Beef liver: 100g contains approximately 14.6 mg of niacin.

Peanuts: 100g provides about 12.8 mg of niacin.

Mushrooms: 100g contains approximately 3.6 mg of niacin.

Green peas: 100g offers around 2.1 mg of niacin.

Brown rice: 100g contains approximately 4.2 mg of niacin.

Vitamin B5 (Pantothenic Acid)

Vitamin B5, also known as pantothenic acid, is a water-soluble vitamin that is essential for the metabolism of carbohydrates, proteins, and fats. It is involved in the production of energy from food and the synthesis of various molecules in the body. Vitamin B5 is sensitive to heat, light, and processing. Therefore, consuming fresh and minimally processed foods can help ensure adequate intake of this vitamin. Deficiency of vitamin B5 is rare, as it is found in a wide variety of foods. Symptoms of deficiency may include fatigue, irritability, numbness or tingling in the hands and feet, and gastrointestinal disturbances.

Recommended Dietary Allowance (RDA): For men and women ages 19 and older is 5 mg daily. For pregnant and lactating women it is 6 mg and 7 mg daily, respectively.

Key functions of vitamin B5 include:

Energy production: Vitamin B5 is a component of coenzyme A (CoA), which is necessary for the breakdown of carbohydrates, proteins, and fats to produce energy.

Hormone synthesis: It plays a role in the synthesis of steroid hormones, such as cortisol, estrogen, and testosterone.

Red blood cell production: Vitamin B5 is involved in the production of red blood cells, which are responsible for carrying oxygen throughout the body.

Skin health: It is believed to have beneficial effects on the skin, helping to maintain its moisture and elasticity. It is often used in skincare products for its moisturizing properties.

Nervous system function: Vitamin B5 is involved in the synthesis of neurotransmitters, which are essential for proper brain function and the transmission of nerve signals.

Immune system support: It helps support the immune system by promoting the production of antibodies and enhancing the function of white blood cells.

Foods sources of Vitamin B5:

Meat: Organ meats, such as liver and kidney, are rich sources of vitamin B5. Other meats like chicken, turkey, and beef also contain pantothenic acid.

Fish: Fish, especially salmon and tuna

Dairy products: Milk, cheese, and yogurt are all sources of vitamin B5. However, the vitamin content may vary depending on the processing and fat content of the dairy product.

Eggs: Eggs are a good source of vitamin B5, particularly the yolk.

Legumes: Lentils, chickpeas, and other legumes contain vitamin B5. They are also a good source of protein and fiber.

Whole grains: Whole grains, such as brown rice, whole wheat bread, and oatmeal, contain vitamin B5. However, refined grains may have lower levels of pantothenic acid due to the removal of the bran and germ.

Nuts and seeds: Nuts, such as peanuts, almonds, and cashews, and seeds, such as sunflower seeds and flaxseeds, contain vitamin B5.

Vegetables: Some vegetables, including broccoli, cauliflower, mushrooms, and sweet potatoes, contain vitamin B5. However, the levels may vary depending on the cooking method and freshness of the vegetables.

Fruits: Fruits like avocados, bananas, and oranges contain small amounts of vitamin B5.

Vitamin B6 (Pyridoxine)

Vitamin B6 is a water-soluble vitamin that plays a crucial role in various bodily functions. It is involved in over 100 enzyme reactions, primarily in the metabolism of amino acids, carbohydrates, and lipids. Deficiency of vitamin B6 is rare but can lead to symptoms such as anemia, skin rashes, depression, confusion, and weakened immune function. Excessive intake of vitamin B6 from supplements can cause nerve damage, so it is important to follow the recommended dosage. Key functions of vitamin B6 include:

Protein metabolism: Vitamin B6 helps in the breakdown and utilization of proteins, ensuring that amino acids are properly metabolized and used for various bodily processes.

Neurotransmitter synthesis: It is involved in the production of neurotransmitters such as serotonin, gamma-aminobutyric acid (GABA) and dopamine, which are important for mood regulation, sleep, and cognitive function.

Red blood cell production: Vitamin B6 is necessary for the synthesis of hemoglobin, the protein responsible for carrying oxygen in red blood cells.

Immune function: It supports the immune system by promoting the production of antibodies and enhancing the activity of white blood cells.

Hormone regulation: Vitamin B6 is involved in the synthesis and metabolism of various hormones, including those involved in the regulation of sleep, mood, and stress response.

Cardiovascular health: It helps in maintaining healthy levels of homocysteine, an amino acid that, when elevated, is associated with an increased risk of cardiovascular diseases.

Recommended Dietary Allowance (RDA): For men and women ages 19 and older is 1.3-1.7 mg daily. For pregnant and lactating women it is 1.9-2.0 mg daily.

Foods sources of Vitamin B6:

Chicken breast: 100g provides about 0.9 mg of Vitamin B6.

Turkey: 100g contains approximately 0.9 mg of Vitamin B6.
Tuna: 100g offers around 0.9 mg of Vitamin B6.
Salmon: 100g provides about 0.9 mg of Vitamin B6.
Pork chops: 100g contains approximately 0.7 mg of Vitamin B6.
Chickpeas: 100g provides about 0.6 mg of Vitamin B6.
Sunflower seeds: 100g contains approximately 1.3 mg of Vitamin B6.
Potatoes: 100g offers around 0.4 mg of Vitamin B6.
Spinach: 100g provides about 0.2 mg of Vitamin B6.
Banana: One medium-sized banana contains approximately 0.4 mg of Vitamin B6.

Vitamin B7 (Biotin)

Vitamin B7, also known as biotin, is a water-soluble vitamin that is part of the B-complex group of vitamins. It plays a crucial role in various metabolic processes in the body. Biotin is involved in the metabolism of carbohydrates, fats, and proteins. It helps convert these macronutrients into energy that the body can use. Biotin also plays a role in the synthesis of fatty acids and the breakdown of amino acids.
One of the well-known functions of biotin is its role in promoting healthy hair, skin, and nails. It is often included in beauty and hair care products due to its potential benefits for maintaining the health and appearance of these tissues.
Biotin is also important for maintaining the health of the nervous system. It is involved in the production of neurotransmitters, which are chemical messengers that allow nerve cells to communicate with each other. Additionally, biotin is necessary for the synthesis of DNA and RNA, the genetic material of cells. It also plays a role in the regulation of gene expression.
Biotin deficiency is rare, as it is found in a wide variety of foods. Good dietary sources of biotin include eggs, nuts, seeds, legumes, whole grains, and certain fruits and vegetables. However, certain conditions or factors, such as pregnancy, long-term antibiotic use, and certain genetic disorders, may increase the risk of biotin deficiency. Supplementation with biotin is sometimes recommended for individuals with certain medical conditions, such as biotinidase deficiency or certain types of hair loss.
Incorporating a variety of biotin-rich foods into your diet can help ensure you're getting an adequate amount of biotin. The Adequate Intake (AI) for biotin for men and women 19 years and older and for pregnant women is 30 micrograms daily. Cooking and processing can affect the biotin content in foods.
Foods sources of Vitamin B7:
Eggs: Egg yolks are a good source of biotin. Eating cooked eggs can provide a significant amount of biotin.

Nuts and seeds: Almonds, walnuts, peanuts, and sunflower seeds are all good sources of biotin. Snacking on these nuts and seeds can help increase your biotin intake.

Legumes: Beans, lentils, and chickpeas are rich in biotin. Including these legumes in your diet can help boost your biotin levels.

Whole grains: Whole grains like oats, brown rice, and barley contain biotin. Opting for whole grain bread, pasta, and cereals can provide you with biotin.

Meat and fish: Organ meats like liver and kidney are high in biotin. Additionally, salmon, tuna, and other types of fish contain biotin. Consuming these meats and fish can contribute to your biotin intake.

Dairy products: Milk, cheese, and yogurt contain biotin. Including these dairy products in your diet can help increase your biotin levels.

Fruits and vegetables: Avocados, bananas, berries, cauliflower, and mushrooms are some fruits and vegetables that contain biotin.

Vitamin B9 (Folic Acid)

Folate, folic acid or vitamin B9, is a water-soluble vitamin that is essential for various functions in the human body. It plays a crucial role in DNA synthesis, red blood cell formation, and the metabolism of amino acids. Folate is also important during periods of rapid growth and development, such as pregnancy.

Folate is naturally found in many foods, including leafy green vegetables, legumes, citrus fruits, and fortified grains. It is also available as a dietary supplement and is often added to processed foods such as bread and breakfast cereals.

During pregnancy, folate is particularly important as it helps in the formation of the neural tube, which develops into the baby's brain and spinal cord.

Adequate folate intake before and during early pregnancy can help reduce the risk of neural tube defects, such as spina bifida, in infants.

Folate deficiency can lead to a condition called folate deficiency anemia, which is characterized by fatigue, weakness, and a decreased ability to produce red blood cells. It may also contribute to an increased risk of certain birth defects and cardiovascular diseases. Cooking methods can affect the folate content in foods. To retain the maximum amount of Vitamin B9, it is recommended to consume these foods raw or lightly cooked.

Recommended Dietary Allowance (RDA): For men and women ages 19 and older is 400-600 micrograms (mcg) of folate daily. Pregnant and lactating women require 600 mcg daily. However, excessive intake of folic acid through supplements can mask a vitamin B12 deficiency, so it is advisable to consult with a healthcare professional for appropriate supplementation.

Foods sources of Vitamin B9:
Leafy greens: Dark leafy greens like spinach, kale, and collard greens are excellent sources of Vitamin B9. They can be consumed raw in salads or cooked in various dishes.
Legumes: Lentils, chickpeas, black beans, and other legumes are high in folate. They can be included in soups, stews, salads, or used as a base for vegetarian dishes.
Asparagus: Asparagus is a versatile vegetable that contains a good amount of Vitamin B9. It can be grilled, roasted, or added to stir-fries and pasta dishes.
Citrus fruits: Citrus fruits such as oranges, lemons, and grapefruits are not only rich in Vitamin C but also provide a decent amount of folate. They can be consumed as whole fruits or used in juices and salads.
Avocado: Avocado is a nutrient-dense fruit that contains various vitamins and minerals, including Vitamin B9. It can be enjoyed sliced on toast, added to salads, or used to make guacamole.
Brussels sprouts: Brussels sprouts are a cruciferous vegetable that is packed with folate. They can be roasted, sautéed, or steamed as a side dish or added to stir-fries.
Sunflower seeds: Sunflower seeds are a good plant-based source of folate. They can be eaten as a snack, sprinkled on salads, or used in baking.
Fortified grains: Many grains, such as bread, pasta, and cereals, are fortified with folic acid, a synthetic form of Vitamin B9. Check the labels to ensure they are fortified.

Vitamin B12 (Cobalamin)

Vitamin B12, also known as cobalamin, is a water-soluble vitamin that is essential for the formation of red blood cells, DNA synthesis, and proper nerve function. It is the only vitamin that contains essential mineral elements. A diet low in B1 and high in folic acid (vegetarian diet) often hides a vitamin B12 deficiency.

B12 is primarily found in animal-based foods such as meat, fish, eggs, and dairy products. It promotes growth and increases appetite in children. It maintains a healthy nervous system improving concentration and memory.
Vitamin B12 deficiency can lead to anemia, neurological problems, and other health issues. In cases of severe vitamin B12 deficiency due to inadequate intrinsic factor (pernicious anemia), doctors may prescribe B12 injections in the muscle.
Recommended Dietary Allowance (RDA): The recommended daily intake of Vitamin B12 for adults is around 2.4 micrograms (mcg). However, these values may vary depending on age, sex, and specific dietary needs.

Vitamin B12 is primarily found in animal-based foods, so it can be more challenging for individuals following a strict vegan or vegetarian diet to obtain adequate amounts of this vitamin. In such cases, fortified foods or supplements may be necessary.
Foods sources of Vitamin B12:
Animal-based sources:
Beef liver: 100g provides about 70.7 mcg of Vitamin B12.
Clams: 100g contains approximately 98.9 mcg of Vitamin B12.
Salmon: 100g offers around 4.9 mcg of Vitamin B12.
Tuna: 100g provides about 2.5 mcg of Vitamin B12.
Chicken: 100g contains approximately 0.3 mcg of Vitamin B12.

Plant-based sources (fortified foods):
Nutritional yeast: 1 tablespoon provides 2.4 mcg of Vitamin B12.
Fortified plant-based milk (such as soy milk or almond milk): 1 cup contains approximately 1-3 mcg of Vitamin B12.
Fortified breakfast cereals: The amount of Vitamin B12 varies, but some brands can provide around 1-6 mcg per serving.

Vitamin C (Ascorbic Acid)

Vitamin C, also known as ascorbic acid, is a water-soluble vitamin that is essential for various bodily functions. It is a powerful antioxidant that helps protect cells from damage caused by free radicals and oxidative stress.
Vitamin C is beneficial for skin health, as it helps protect against sun damage, promotes collagen synthesis, and reduces the appearance of wrinkles and fine lines. Deficiency of vitamin C can lead to a condition called scurvy, characterized by fatigue, weakness, joint pain, bleeding gums, and impaired wound healing. Excessive intake of vitamin C from supplements can cause digestive issues, such as diarrhea and stomach cramps. It is important to follow the recommended dosage and consult with a healthcare professional before starting any new supplement regimen.
The vitamin C content in foods can vary depending on factors such as ripeness, cooking methods, and storage conditions.
Recommended Dietary Allowance (RDA): The recommended daily intake of vitamin C varies depending on age, sex, and life stage, but generally is 90 mg daily for men and 75 mg for women. For pregnant women is 85 mg and 120 mg for lactating women 120 mg daily.
Key functions of vitamin C include:
Immune function: Vitamin C plays a crucial role in supporting the immune system. It helps stimulate the production of white blood cells, which are important for fighting off

infections and pathogens. It also enhances the function of immune cells and promotes the production of antibodies.

Collagen synthesis: Vitamin C is necessary for the synthesis of collagen, a protein that provides structure and strength to connective tissues, such as skin, bones, and blood vessels. It is essential for wound healing, tissue repair, and maintaining healthy skin.

Antioxidant activity: Vitamin C acts as a potent antioxidant, neutralizing harmful free radicals and protecting cells from oxidative damage. It also regenerates other antioxidants, such as vitamin E, and enhances their effectiveness.

Iron absorption: Vitamin C enhances the absorption of non-heme iron, the type of iron found in plant-based foods. It helps convert iron into a more absorbable form, increasing its uptake in the intestines.

Neurotransmitter synthesis: Vitamin C is involved in the synthesis of neurotransmitters, such as serotonin and norepinephrine, which are important for mood regulation and cognitive function.

Foods sources of Vitamin C:

Citrus Fruits: Oranges, lemons, limes, and grapefruits are excellent sources of vitamin C. One medium-sized orange provides about 70-90 mg of vitamin C.

Berries: Strawberries, blueberries, raspberries, and blackberries are all rich in vitamin C. For example, one cup of strawberries contains approximately 85 mg of vitamin C.

Kiwi: This small fruit is packed with vitamin C. One medium-sized kiwi provides around 70-90 mg of vitamin C.

Papaya: A medium-sized papaya contains about 90 mg of vitamin C.

Pineapple: This tropical fruit is not only delicious but also a good source of vitamin C. One cup of pineapple chunks contains approximately 8090 mg of vitamin C.

Mango: Another tropical fruit, one medium-sized mango provides around 60-70 mg of vitamin C.

Bell Peppers: Red, yellow, and green bell peppers are all high in vitamin C. One medium-sized bell pepper can provide anywhere from 95-150 mg of vitamin C, with red peppers generally having the highest content.

Leafy Greens: Vegetables like kale, spinach, and Swiss chard contain vitamin C. For example, one cup of cooked kale contains about 80 mg of vitamin C.

Tomatoes: These juicy fruits are a good source of vitamin C. One medium-sized tomato provides around 30 mg of vitamin C.

Broccoli: This cruciferous vegetable is not only rich in various nutrients but also contains vitamin C. One cup of cooked broccoli contains approximately 80 mg of vitamin C.

Vitamin D (calciferol)

Vitamin D is a fat-soluble vitamin that is essential for the body's overall health and well-being. It plays a crucial role in the absorption of calcium and phosphorus, which are important for maintaining strong bones and teeth.

Vitamin D can be obtained through exposure to sunlight, as the skin produces it when exposed to UVB rays. It can also be obtained through certain foods, such as fatty fish (salmon, mackerel, sardines), fortified dairy products, egg yolks, and mushrooms.

In addition to its role in bone health, vitamin D also plays a role in immune function, muscle function, and cell growth. It has been linked to a reduced risk of certain diseases, such as osteoporosis, heart disease, and certain types of cancer.

Deficiency in vitamin D can lead to various health problems, including rickets in children and osteomalacia in adults, which are characterized by weak and brittle bones. Symptoms of deficiency may also include fatigue, muscle weakness, bone pain, and a weakened immune system.

It is recommended that most adults get at least 600-800 international units (IU) of vitamin D per day, although individual needs may vary. Some people may require higher doses, especially those with limited sun exposure, darker skin, or certain medical conditions. Excessive intake of vitamin D can lead to toxicity, which can cause symptoms such as nausea, vomiting, poor appetite, constipation, weakness, and kidney problems. It is important to not exceed the recommended daily intake without medical supervision. Maintaining adequate levels of vitamin D is important for overall health and well-being, and it is recommended to obtain it through a combination of sunlight exposure, dietary sources, and supplements if necessary.

Vitamin D is primarily synthesized in the body through exposure to sunlight. However, getting enough sunlight can be challenging, especially in certain seasons or for individuals living in northern latitudes. In such cases, incorporating vitamin D-rich foods into your diet can help meet your needs.

Foods sources of Vitamin D:

Fatty Fish: Fatty fish like salmon, trout, mackerel, and sardines are excellent sources of vitamin D. For example, a 3.5-ounce serving of cooked salmon can provide around 400-600 IU (International Units) of vitamin D.

Cod Liver Oil: This oil is derived from the liver of cod fish and is one of the richest sources of vitamin D. Just one tablespoon of cod liver oil can provide around 1,300-1,400 IU of vitamin D.

Canned Tuna: Tuna, especially canned in oil, is a good source of vitamin D. A 3.5-ounce serving of canned tuna can provide approximately 150-200 IU of vitamin D.

Egg Yolks: Egg yolks contain small amounts of vitamin D. One large egg yolk provides around 40 IU of vitamin D.

Cheese: Some types of cheese, such as Swiss cheese, cheddar cheese, and mozzarella, contain small amounts of vitamin D. It is generally around 1-6 IU per ounce.

Mushrooms: Certain types of mushrooms, such as shiitake and maitake mushrooms, can provide vitamin D when exposed to ultraviolet (UV) light. The amount can vary, but it is typically around 100-400 IU per 3.5 ounces of mushrooms.

Fortified Foods: Many foods are fortified with vitamin D to help increase intake. This includes fortified milk, orange juice, breakfast cereals, and plant-based milk alternatives. The amount of vitamin D can vary depending on the product, so it's important to check the labels.

Vitamin E (tocopherols)

Vitamin E is a fat-soluble vitamin that acts as an antioxidant in the body. It helps protect cells from damage caused by free radicals, which are unstable molecules that can harm cells and contribute to chronic diseases.

In addition to its antioxidant properties, vitamin E plays a role in immune function, cell signaling, and gene expression.

It also helps in the formation of red blood cells and the maintenance of healthy skin and eyes.

There is some evidence to suggest that vitamin E may have potential health benefits, such as reducing the risk of heart disease, certain types of cancer, and age-related macular degeneration.

The vitamin E content in foods can vary depending on factors such as processing, storage, and cooking methods. Additionally, vitamin E is a fat-soluble vitamin, so consuming it with a source of healthy fats can enhance its absorption.

Recommended Dietary Allowance (RDA): The recommended daily intake of vitamin E for adults is 15 milligrams (or 22.4 international units) per day. Lactating women need slightly more at 19 mg (28 IU) daily.

Most people can easily meet their vitamin E needs through a balanced diet, but supplementation may be necessary for individuals with certain medical conditions or those who have difficulty absorbing fat.

Excessive intake of vitamin E through supplements can have adverse effects, such as an increased risk of bleeding. Therefore, it is generally recommended to obtain vitamin E from food sources rather than relying solely on supplements.

Foods sources of Vitamin E:

Nuts and Seeds: Many nuts and seeds are rich in vitamin E. Almonds, sunflower seeds, hazelnuts, and peanuts are particularly high in vitamin E. For example, one ounce (28 grams) of almonds provides around 7.3 mg of vitamin E.

Spinach and Other Leafy Greens: Leafy greens like spinach, Swiss chard, and kale contain vitamin E. For instance, one cup of cooked spinach provides approximately 3.7 mg of vitamin E.

Olive Oil: Olive oil is a good source of vitamin E, particularly when consumed in its extra virgin form.

The vitamin E content in olive oil can vary depending on the type of olive oil and its processing. Extra virgin olive oil, which is the least processed and retains more of the natural nutrients, including vitamin E, can contain around 1.9 milligrams of vitamin E per tablespoon (13.5 grams) of oil.

Other types of olive oil, such as virgin or regular olive oil, may have slightly lower vitamin E content due to more processing.

Vegetable Oils: Certain vegetable oils are good sources of vitamin E.

Wheat germ oil, sunflower oil, and safflower oil are particularly high in vitamin E. Just one tablespoon of wheat germ oil can provide around 20.3 mg of vitamin E.

Avocado: Avocado is a fruit that is rich in healthy fats and vitamin E. One medium-sized avocado contains approximately 2.7 mg of vitamin E.

Mango: This tropical fruit is not only delicious but also contains vitamin E. One medium-sized mango provides around 1.8 mg of vitamin E.

Red Bell Peppers: Red bell peppers are a good source of vitamin E. One medium-sized red bell pepper provides approximately 1.9 mg of vitamin E.

Broccoli: This cruciferous vegetable contains vitamin E. One cup of cooked broccoli contains approximately 1.2 mg of vitamin E.

Tomatoes: Tomatoes are a source of vitamin E. One medium-sized tomato contains around 0.7 mg of vitamin E.

Whole Grains: Whole grains like wheat germ, brown rice, and oats contain vitamin E. The exact amount can vary, but it is generally around 0.5-2 mg per serving.

Vitamin K

Vitamin K is a fat-soluble vitamin that plays a crucial role in blood clotting and bone health.

There are two main forms of vitamin K: vitamin K1 (phylloquinone) and vitamin K2 (menaquinone).

Vitamin K1 is involved in the production of clotting factors in the liver, which are necessary for the blood to clot properly. Without sufficient vitamin K1, a person may experience excessive bleeding or bruising.

Vitamin K2, on the other hand, is produced by bacteria in the gut and is also found in certain animal products and fermented foods. It is involved in regulating calcium metabolism and promoting bone health. Vitamin K2 helps to activate proteins that direct calcium to the bones and teeth, preventing it from accumulating in the arteries and soft tissues.

In addition to its role in blood clotting and bone health, vitamin K may also have other health benefits. Some studies suggest that it may help reduce the risk of heart disease, improve insulin sensitivity, and support brain function. However, more research is needed to fully understand these potential benefits.

The recommended daily intake of vitamin K varies depending on age and gender. For adults, the recommended daily intake is 90-120 micrograms for men and 90 micrograms for women. Excessive intake of vitamin K through supplements can interfere with certain medications, such as blood thinners, so it is always best to consult with a healthcare professional before starting any new supplements.

Vitamin K is a fat-soluble vitamin, so consuming it with a source of healthy fats can enhance its absorption. Vitamin K plays a crucial role in blood clotting.

Individuals taking blood-thinning medications should consult with their healthcare provider before making significant changes to their vitamin K intake.

Foods sources of Vitamin K:

Leafy Greens: Kale, spinach, Swiss chard, collard greens, and mustard greens contain vitamin K. For instance, one cup of cooked kale provides around 1062 micrograms (mcg) of vitamin K.

Cruciferous Vegetables: Cruciferous vegetables like broccoli, Brussels sprouts, and cabbage also contain vitamin K. One cup of cooked broccoli provides around 220 mcg of vitamin K.

Herbs: Fresh herbs like parsley, basil, oregano and cilantro are good sources of vitamin K. For example, one tablespoon of fresh parsley contains approximately 82 mcg of vitamin K and just two teaspoons of oregano will meet a significant percentage of your daily Vitamin K needs. On average, one tablespoon (around 2 grams) of fresh basil contains approximately 32 micrograms of vitamin K.

Green Peas: Green peas contain vitamin K. One cup of cooked green peas provides around 24 mcg of vitamin K.

Green Beans: Green beans are another vegetable that contains vitamin K. One cup of cooked green beans provides approximately 14 mcg of vitamin K.

Brussels Sprouts: Brussels sprouts are a cruciferous vegetable that contains vitamin K. One cup of cooked Brussels sprouts provides around 218 mcg of vitamin K.

Asparagus: Asparagus is a vegetable that contains vitamin K. One cup of cooked asparagus provides 55 mcg of vitamin K.

Avocado: Avocado is a fruit that contains small amounts of vitamin K. One medium-sized avocado provides around 21 mcg of vitamin K.

Prunes: Prunes, also known as dried plums, are a fruit that contains vitamin K. One cup of prunes provides approximately 60 mcg of vitamin K.

Minerals

The essential minerals in the human body include calcium, phosphorus, magnesium, sodium, potassium, chloride, iron, zinc, copper, manganese, iodine, selenium, and molybdenum. These minerals are required in small amounts for various physiological processes and functions in the body. While these minerals are vital for health, they should be consumed in appropriate amounts. Excessive intake of certain minerals can be harmful.

Calcium

Calcium is a chemical element with the symbol Ca and atomic number 20. It is a soft gray alkaline earth metal and is the fifth-most abundant element by mass in the Earth's crust and the most abundant in the human body. Calcium is essential for living organisms, as it plays a crucial role in various biological processes. It is particularly important for the formation and maintenance of strong bones and teeth. Calcium also plays a role in muscle contraction, nerve function, blood clotting, and cell signaling. It is commonly found in dairy products, leafy green vegetables, and fortified foods. The calcium content in foods can vary depending on factors such as processing, cooking methods, and storage conditions. It is important to consume calcium-rich foods in combination with adequate vitamin D intake, as vitamin D helps with calcium absorption.

Foods sources of Calcium:
Dairy Products: Dairy products like milk, cheese, and yogurt are excellent sources of calcium. For example, one cup of milk provides around 300 mg of calcium.
Leafy Greens: Leafy green vegetables like kale, spinach, and collard greens contain calcium. One cup of cooked kale provides approximately 94 mg of calcium.
Tofu: Tofu, made from soybeans, is a good source of calcium. The exact amount can vary depending on the brand and type, but it is generally around 150-250 mg per half cup.
Canned Fish with Bones: Canned fish like salmon and sardines, when consumed with the bones, are rich in calcium. One can of salmon with bones provides around 300-400 mg of calcium.
Fortified Plant-Based Milk Alternatives: Many plant-based milk alternatives, such as almond milk, soy milk, and oat milk, are fortified with calcium.
Fortified Breakfast Cereals: Some breakfast cereals are fortified with calcium. The amount can vary depending on the brand and type, so it's important to check the labels.

Beans and Legumes: Certain beans and legumes, such as white beans, chickpeas, and black-eyed peas, contain calcium. One cup of cooked white beans provides approximately 160 mg of calcium.

Nuts and Seeds: Some nuts and seeds, such as almonds, sesame seeds, and chia seeds, contain calcium. For instance, one ounce of almonds provides around 75 mg of calcium.

Fortified Orange Juice: Some brands of orange juice are fortified with calcium. The amount can vary depending on the brand, so it is important to check the labels.

Amaranth and Quinoa: These pseudo-grains are good sources of calcium. For example, one cup of cooked amaranth (246 grams) provides approximately 116 milligrams of calcium and a cup of cooked quinoa (185 grams) provides approximately 31 milligrams of calcium.

Phosphorus

Phosphorus is an essential mineral in the human body that plays a crucial role in many physiological processes. It is a key component of DNA, RNA, and ATP, which are essential molecules for cell function and energy production. Phosphorus is also important for bone health, as it is a major component of hydroxyapatite, the mineral complex that provides strength and structure to bones and teeth. This mineral works with calcium to build strong bones and teeth. Additionally, phosphorus is involved in the regulation of acid-base balance, the formation of cell membranes, and the production of hormones.

Foods sources of phosphorus:

Dairy products: Milk, yogurt, and cheese are rich sources of phosphorus.
  - Milk (1 cup): 247 mg
  - Yogurt (1 cup): 385 mg
  - Cheese (1 oz): 120-200 mg

Meat and poultry: Beef, pork, chicken, and turkey are good sources of phosphorus.
  - Beef (3 oz): 220 mg
  - Pork (3 oz): 250 mg
  - Chicken (3 oz): 200 mg
  - Turkey (3 oz): 230 mg

Seafood: Fish, shellfish, and other seafood are high in phosphorus.
  - Salmon (3 oz): 270 mg
  - Shrimp (3 oz): 200 mg
  - Tuna (3 oz): 200 mg

Nuts and seeds: Almonds, sunflower seeds, and pumpkin seeds are good sources of phosphorus.
  - Almonds (1 oz): 135 mg

- Sunflower seeds (1 oz): 150 mg
- Pumpkin seeds (1 oz): 225 mg

Legumes: Lentils, chickpeas, and beans are rich in phosphorus.
- Lentils (1 cup): 356 mg
- Chickpeas (1 cup): 282 mg
- Black beans (1 cup): 241 mg

Whole grains: Whole wheat, brown rice, and quinoa are good sources of phosphorus.
- Whole wheat bread (1 slice): 25 mg
- Brown rice (1 cup): 150 mg
- Quinoa (1 cup): 281 mg

Eggs: Eggs are a good source of phosphorus.
- Egg (1 large): 96 mg

Fruits and vegetables: Some fruits and vegetables, such as potatoes, broccoli, and oranges, also contain phosphorus.
- Potato (1 medium): 121 mg
- Broccoli (1 cup): 50 mg
- Orange (1 medium): 13 mg

Iron

Iron is a chemical element with the symbol Fe and atomic number 26. It is a lustrous, silvery-gray metal that is abundant in the Earth's crust. Iron is an essential element for living organisms, as it plays a crucial role in various biological processes. It is a key component of hemoglobin, a protein in red blood cells that carries oxygen from the lungs to the rest of the body. Iron is also essential for the production of myoglobin, a protein that helps muscles store and use oxygen. Additionally, iron is involved in energy production, immune function, and DNA synthesis.

It is important to consume an adequate amount of iron through diet to maintain optimal health. Iron deficiency can lead to anemia, fatigue, and impaired cognitive function. It is important to consume iron-rich foods along with sources of vitamin C (such as citrus fruits, strawberries, and bell peppers) to enhance iron absorption. Additionally, cooking in cast-iron cookware can increase the iron content of your meals.

Foods that are good sources of iron include:

Red meat: Beef, lamb, and pork are rich sources of heme iron, which is more easily absorbed by the body.
- Beef (3 oz): 2.3 mg of iron
- Lamb (3 oz): 1.2 mg of iron

- Pork (3 oz): 0.9 mg of iron

Poultry: Chicken and turkey are good sources of heme iron.
- Chicken (3 oz): 1.1 mg of iron
- Turkey (3 oz): 0.9 mg of iron

Seafood: Shellfish, such as oysters and clams, are rich in iron.
- Oysters (3 oz): 7.2 mg of iron
- Clams (3 oz): 2.3 mg of iron

Beans and legumes: Lentils, chickpeas, and kidney beans are good sources of non-heme iron.
- Lentils (1 cup): 6.6 mg of iron
- Chickpeas (1 cup): 4.7 mg of iron
- Kidney beans (1 cup): 3.9 mg of iron

Nuts and seeds: Pumpkin seeds, cashews, and almonds are rich in iron.
- Pumpkin seeds (1 oz): 4.2 mg of iron
- Cashews (1 oz): 1.7 mg of iron
- Almonds (1 oz): 1.0 mg of iron

Whole grains: Quinoa, oats, and brown rice are rich in iron.
- Quinoa (1 cup, cooked): 2.8 mg
- Oats (1 cup, cooked): 3.4 mg
- Brown rice (1 cup, cooked): 0.8 mg

Fortified cereals: Many breakfast cereals are fortified with iron.
- Fortified cereal (1 cup): varies, typically around 18 mg of iron

Dark leafy greens: Spinach, kale, and Swiss chard are good sources of non-heme iron.
- Spinach (1 cup): 6.4 mg of iron
- Collard greens (1 cup, cooked): 2.2 mg
- Kale (1 cup): 1.1 mg of iron
- Swiss chard (1 cup): 0.6 mg of iron

Dried fruits: Raisins, apricots, prunes, and dates are dried fruits that are good sources of iron. Dried fruits are a convenient and portable snack option that can provide a source of iron and other nutrients. They can be added to oatmeal, yogurt, salads, or eaten on their own as a healthy snack.
- Raisins (1/2 cup, packed): 1.1 mg
- Apricots, dried (1/2 cup): 1.3 mg
- Prunes (dried plums, 1/2 cup, pitted): 1.4 mg
- Dates (pitted, 1/2 cup): 1.2 mg

Tofu: Made from soybeans, tofu is a vegetarian source of iron. Tofu, also known as bean curd, is a popular plant-based protein source that is made from soybeans. Tofu is a good source of non-heme iron, which is the type of iron found in plant-based foods. In addition to iron, tofu is also rich in protein, calcium, and other nutrients.

Incorporating tofu into your meals can help boost your iron intake, especially if you follow a vegetarian or vegan diet.
   - Tofu (1/2 cup, firm):
   - Iron content: 6.6 mg
Dark chocolate: Dark chocolate with a high cocoa content (70% or higher) is a better source of iron compared to milk chocolate. While dark chocolate can contribute to your iron intake, it is important to consume it in moderation due to its calorie and sugar content. Enjoying a small amount of dark chocolate as an occasional treat can be a tasty way to add some iron to your diet.
Dark chocolate (1 oz): Iron content: 3.3 mg

Magnesium

Magnesium is a chemical element with the symbol Mg and atomic number 12. It is a shiny gray metal that is abundant in the Earth's crust.
Magnesium is an essential mineral for living organisms, as it plays a crucial role in various biological processes. It is involved in over 300 enzymatic reactions in the body, including energy production, protein synthesis, muscle and nerve function, and DNA synthesis. Magnesium also helps regulate blood pressure, maintain a steady heart rhythm, and support bone health.
It is commonly found in nuts, seeds, whole grains, leafy green vegetables, and legumes. Magnesium deficiency can lead to muscle weakness, fatigue, and abnormal heart rhythms.
The magnesium content of foods can vary depending on factors such as soil quality and processing methods. Aim to include a variety of these magnesium-rich foods in your diet to ensure an adequate intake of this essential mineral.
Foods sources of magnesium include:
Legumes: Beans, lentils, chickpeas, green peas and soybeans are not only high in magnesium but also provide other essential nutrients like protein, fiber and vitamins.
   - Soybeans (1 cup, cooked):148 mg of Magnesium
   - Black beans (1 cup, cooked): 120 mg of magnesium
   - Chickpeas (1 cup, cooked): 78 mg of magnesium
   - Lentils (1 cup, cooked): 71 mg of magnesium
   - Green peas (1 cup, cooked): 46 mg of Magnesium
Whole grains: Whole wheat, brown rice, quinoa, oats, and barley are examples of whole grains that contain magnesium.
   - Whole wheat flour (1 cup): 176 mg of Magnesium
   - Quinoa (1 cup, cooked): 118 mg of magnesium
   - Brown rice (1 cup, cooked): 86 mg of magnesium

- Oats (1 cup, cooked): 61 mg of magnesium
- Barley (1 cup, cooked): 55 mg of magnesium

Dark leafy greens: Spinach, kale, Swiss chard, and collard greens are not only packed with iron but also provide a good amount of magnesium.
- Spinach (1 cup, cooked): 157 mg of magnesium
- Swiss chard (1 cup, cooked): 150 mg of magnesium
- Collard greens (1 cup, cooked): 39 mg of Magnesium
- Kale (1 cup, cooked): 23 mg of magnesium

Fatty fish: Fish like mackerel, halibut, sardines, anchovies and salmon are not only rich in omega-3 fatty acids but also provide magnesium and other nutrients like protein, and calcium.
- Mackerel (3 oz): 97 mg of magnesium
- Halibut (3 oz): 90 mg of magnesium
- Sardines (3 oz): 42 mg of magnesium
- Anchovies (3 oz): 38 mg of magnesium
- Salmon (3 oz): 26 mg of magnesium

Nuts and seeds: Almonds, cashews, peanuts, pumpkin seeds, and sesame seeds are all rich in magnesium.
- Pumpkin seeds (1 oz): 150 mg
- Almonds (1 oz): 80 mg of magnesium
- Cashews (1 oz): 74 mg of magnesium
- Peanuts (1 oz): 50 mg of magnesium
- Sesame seeds (1 oz): 101 mg

Avocado: This creamy fruit is a good source of magnesium, along with healthy fats and fiber.
- Avocado (1 medium): 58 mg of magnesium

Bananas: In addition to being a good source of potassium, bananas also contain magnesium.
- Banana (1 medium): 32 mg of magnesium

Dark chocolate (70-85% cocoa): Dark chocolate with a high cocoa content is not only a delicious treat but also provides magnesium.
- Dark chocolate (1 oz): 64 mg of magnesium

Yogurt: Plain yogurt is a good source of magnesium, along with calcium and probiotics. Including yogurt in your diet can help increase your magnesium intake and support gut health, bone health, and overall well-being.
- Plain yogurt (1 cup): 47 mg of magnesium

Tofu: Made from soybeans, tofu is a vegetarian source of magnesium. Tofu is a plant-based source of magnesium and is also rich in protein, iron, and calcium.
- Firm tofu (1/2 cup, raw): Magnesium content: 81 mg

Potassium

Potassium is an essential mineral and electrolyte that plays a vital role in various physiological processes in the human body. It is classified as an alkali metal and has the atomic number 19 and the symbol K.

Potassium is primarily found inside cells, and it helps maintain proper cell function, nerve transmission, and muscle contraction. It is also involved in maintaining fluid balance, regulating blood pressure, and supporting heart health.

A deficiency in potassium, known as hypokalemia, can occur due to factors such as inadequate dietary intake, excessive fluid loss (e.g., through sweating or diarrhea), or certain medical conditions. Symptoms of potassium deficiency may include muscle weakness, fatigue, cramps, irregular heartbeat, and constipation.

On the other hand, excessive potassium intake, known as hyperkalemia, can also be problematic and may occur in individuals with kidney problems or those taking certain medications. High levels of potassium can disrupt the normal electrical activity of the heart and lead to irregular heart rhythms.

The recommended daily intake of potassium for adults is around 2,600-3,400 milligrams, although individual requirements may vary. It is generally advisable to obtain potassium from a balanced diet rather than relying solely on supplements, unless specifically recommended by a healthcare professional.

Foods sources of Potassium:

Spinach: Leafy greens like spinach are not only rich in iron and magnesium but also provide a good amount of potassium.
100 grams = 558 mg

Bananas: Bananas are well-known for their potassium content. They are a convenient and portable snack option.
100 grams = 358 mg

Avocado: Avocados are not only rich in healthy fats but also provide a good amount of potassium.
100 grams = 485 mg

Sweet potatoes: Sweet potatoes are a nutritious root vegetable that is high in potassium, fiber, and other essential nutrients.
100 grams = 337 mg

White beans: White beans, such as cannellini beans, are one of the best sources of potassium among legumes.
100 grams = 561 mg

Salmon: Fatty fish like salmon are not only a good source of omega-3 fatty acids but also provide potassium.
100 grams = 628 mg
Yogurt: Plain yogurt is a good source of potassium, along with calcium and probiotics. A cup of plain yogurt (approximately 245 grams) contains about 380 milligrams of potassium. This may vary slightly depending on the brand and type (such as low-fat, non-fat, or whole milk).
Tomatoes: Tomatoes are not only a versatile ingredient but also provide potassium, along with other vitamins and minerals. A medium-sized raw tomato (about 123 grams) contains approximately 292 milligrams of potassium.
Oranges: Oranges and other citrus fruits like grapefruits and tangerines are not only high in vitamin C but also provide potassium. The potassium content can vary slightly based on the size of the fruit and its ripeness.
- Orange: A medium-sized orange (approximately 131 grams) has about 237 milligrams of potassium.
- Grapefruit: A half of a medium-sized grapefruit (123 grams) contains about 166 milligrams of potassium.
- Tangerine: A medium-sized tangerine (about 88 grams) contains about 132 milligrams of potassium.

Coconut water: Coconut water is a natural source of potassium and is often consumed as a hydrating beverage. One cup of coconut water (about 240 grams) contains approximately 600 milligrams of potassium. This can vary slightly depending on the brand and freshness of the coconut water.

Potassium requirements can vary depending on factors such as age, sex, and overall health. The actual potassium content of foods can vary, depending on factors such as soil composition and processing methods.

Chloride

Chloride is an essential mineral and an electrolyte that plays a crucial role in maintaining the balance of fluids in the body. Chloride is mainly found in the extracellular fluid, which includes the fluid outside the cells.

Functions of Chloride in the body:

Fluid Balance: Chloride works together with sodium to maintain the balance of fluids in the body. It helps regulate the movement of water in and out of cells, ensuring proper hydration.

Acid-Base Balance: Chloride is involved in maintaining the pH balance of body fluids. It helps in the production of stomach acid, which aids in digestion.

Nerve Function: Chloride is essential for the transmission of nerve impulses and muscle function. It plays a role in the movement of electrical signals across cell membranes.

Digestion: Chloride is involved in the production of hydrochloric acid in the stomach, which is necessary for the breakdown of food and absorption of nutrients.

Immune Function: Chloride plays a role in the immune response of the body, helping to fight off infections and maintain overall immune function.

Chloride is obtained through the diet, primarily from table salt (sodium chloride) and other salty foods. It is also present in smaller amounts in foods like seaweed, celery, tomatoes, and olives. The recommended daily intake of chloride for adults is around 2300-3400 mg.

Sodium

Sodium is a chemical element with the symbol Na and atomic number 11. It is a soft, silvery-white, highly reactive metal and is a member of the alkali metal group of elements. Sodium is found in many minerals, such as halite (rock salt) and soda ash, and is essential for various biological processes in humans and other animals. It plays a crucial role in maintaining fluid balance, transmitting nerve impulses, and contracting muscles. Sodium is also widely used in industry, particularly in the production of chemicals, glass, and metals.

Sodium is essential for human health, but it is important to consume it in moderation. It plays a crucial role in maintaining fluid balance, transmitting nerve impulses, and contracting muscles. Sodium helps regulate blood pressure and volume, and it is involved in the functioning of the kidneys and adrenal glands. However, excessive sodium intake can have negative effects on health. High sodium consumption is associated with an increased risk of high blood pressure, which in turn can lead to heart disease, stroke, and other cardiovascular problems. It can also contribute to the development of kidney disease and osteoporosis.

The recommended daily intake of sodium for adults is generally around 2,300 milligrams (mg), but this can vary depending on individual health conditions. It is important to be mindful of sodium intake and to consume a balanced diet that includes a variety of foods, including fruits, vegetables, whole grains, and lean proteins, to ensure adequate nutrition while minimizing excessive sodium intake.

While sodium is an essential mineral, excessive intake can contribute to high blood pressure and other health issues. It is recommended to consume sodium in moderation and choose lower-sodium options when possible.

Foods sources of Sodium:

Table salt: Table salt, also known as sodium chloride, is the most common source of sodium in the diet. It is used as a seasoning in cooking and added to many processed foods.

Processed meats: Deli meats, bacon, sausage, and hot dogs are often high in sodium due to the curing and preserving processes.

Canned soups and broths: Canned soups and broths can be high in sodium, so it's important to check the labels and choose low-sodium options when available.

Condiments and sauces: Condiments like soy sauce, ketchup, barbecue sauce, and salad dressings can contain significant amounts of sodium.

Cheese: Some types of cheese, especially processed cheese and certain varieties like feta and blue cheese, can be high in sodium.

Pickles and olives: Pickles and olives are often brined in a salty solution, making them a source of sodium.

Snack foods: Chips, pretzels, popcorn, and other snack foods are often seasoned with salt and can be high in sodium.

Fast food and restaurant meals: Many fast food and restaurant meals are high in sodium due to the use of processed ingredients and added salt.

Bread and baked goods: Some bread and baked goods, especially those made with processed flours, can contain added salt.

Canned vegetables: Canned vegetables may contain added salt as a preservative, so it's important to choose low-sodium or no-salt-added options.

Sea salt and iodized salt are considered sources of sodium. Sodium chloride is the main component of both types of salt, and it is the sodium in sodium chloride that is of concern when it comes to dietary sodium intake.

Sea salt is derived from evaporated seawater and may contain trace amounts of other minerals, giving it a slightly different flavor and appearance compared to table salt. Iodized salt, on the other hand, is table salt that has been fortified with iodine, an essential nutrient for thyroid function.

Regardless of the type of salt, it is important to consume sodium in moderation as excessive sodium intake can have negative health effects, such as high blood pressure.

Both sea salt and iodized salt have their own advantages and considerations. Key points to consider:

Iodine content: Iodized salt is fortified with iodine, an essential mineral that is important for thyroid function and the production of thyroid hormones. Sea salt, on the other hand, generally does not contain significant amounts of iodine. If you have a low iodine intake or live in an area with iodine deficiency, iodized salt may be a better choice to ensure adequate iodine levels.

Mineral content: Sea salt is often touted for its natural mineral content, which can include trace amounts of minerals like magnesium, calcium, and potassium. However, the amounts of these minerals in sea salt are typically very small and may not have a significant impact on overall nutrition.

Processing: Iodized salt undergoes a process where iodine is added to the salt crystals. Sea salt is typically less processed and may contain fewer additives or anti-caking agents. Some people prefer the more natural and less processed nature of sea salt.

Taste and texture: Sea salt is known for its larger, coarser crystals and can have a more distinct flavor compared to iodized salt. The taste and texture of salt can vary depending on the source and processing methods.

Ultimately, the choice between sea salt and iodized salt depends on individual preferences, dietary needs, and health considerations.

Zinc

Zinc is a chemical element with the symbol Zn and atomic number 30. It is a bluish-white metal that is commonly used in various industries due to its unique properties. Zinc is found in the Earth's crust and is the 24th most abundant element. Zinc has been used by humans for thousands of years. Ancient civilizations, such as the Romans and Greeks, used zinc for various purposes, including making brass and as a medicinal ingredient. The element was first recognized as a distinct metal in the 16th century. Major zinc-producing countries include China, Australia, Peru, and the United States. Zinc is highly recyclable, and the recycling process consumes significantly less energy compared to primary production. Recycling zinc helps conserve natural resources and reduces environmental impact.

Zinc is a versatile element with a wide range of applications in various industries. Its unique properties and health benefits make it an essential element for both industrial and biological purposes. The zinc content can vary depending on factors such as soil quality, processing methods, and cooking techniques.

Key facts about zinc:

Health benefits: Zinc plays a crucial role in various biological processes in the human body. It is essential for proper immune function, wound healing, and DNA synthesis.

Zinc supplements are often used to treat zinc deficiency, which can lead to impaired growth, weakened immune system, and other health issues.

Hazards: While zinc is generally considered safe for humans, excessive intake can lead to adverse effects, such as nausea, vomiting, and diarrhea. Prolonged exposure to high levels of zinc can also cause respiratory issues and damage to the nervous system.

Foods sources of Zinc:

Shellfish: Oysters are the richest source of zinc, with about 74 mg per 100 grams. Other shellfish like crab, lobster, and mussels also contain significant amounts of zinc.

Meat: Beef and lamb are good sources of zinc, with around 4-5 mg per 100 grams. Pork and chicken also contain smaller amounts of zinc.

Legumes: Chickpeas, lentils, and beans like black beans and kidney beans are all good sources of zinc. They typically contain around 2-3 mg per 100 grams.

Nuts and seeds: Pumpkin seeds (also known as pepitas) are particularly high in zinc, with about 7-8 mg per 100 grams. Other nuts and seeds like cashews, almonds, and sesame seeds also contain zinc.

Dairy products: Milk and cheese are moderate sources of zinc, with around 1-2 mg per 100 grams. Yogurt and other dairy products also contain smaller amounts of zinc.

Whole grains: Whole grains like wheat, oats, and quinoa contain zinc, although the amounts are relatively small compared to other sources. They typically provide around 1-2 mg per 100 grams.

Vegetables: Some vegetables like spinach, kale, and mushrooms contain small amounts of zinc. However, the bioavailability of zinc from plant-based sources is generally lower compared to animal-based sources.

Copper

Copper is a chemical element with the symbol Cu and atomic number 29. It is a reddish-brown metal that has been used by humans for thousands of years. Copper is a trace mineral in the human body, meaning it is present in very small amounts. The human body contains about 1.4 to 2.1 mg of copper per kilogram of body weight. So, for a person weighing 70 kilograms (about 154 pounds), this would equate to approximately 98 to 147 milligrams of copper in total in the body. This is about 0.000015% of the total body weight. Copper is essential for various bodily functions including iron transport, energy metabolism, and brain function. It is also a part of several enzymes.

Key facts about copper and its benefits to the human body:
Essential nutrient: Copper is an essential trace mineral that is required for the proper functioning of the human body. It plays a crucial role in various biological processes, including the formation of red blood cells, maintenance of connective tissues, and functioning of the immune system.
Antioxidant properties: Copper acts as an antioxidant in the body, helping to neutralize harmful free radicals and reduce oxidative stress. This can help protect cells and tissues from damage and may have anti-aging effects.
Iron absorption: Copper is necessary for the absorption and utilization of iron in the body. It helps convert iron into a form that can be easily absorbed by the intestines and transported to various tissues. Adequate copper levels are important for preventing iron deficiency anemia.
Energy production: Copper is involved in the production of adenosine triphosphate (ATP), which is the primary source of energy for cells. It is a cofactor for enzymes involved in energy metabolism, including those responsible for the production of ATP in the mitochondria.
Connective tissue health: Copper is essential for the synthesis and maintenance of connective tissues, such as collagen and elastin. These tissues provide structure and support to various organs, including the skin, blood vessels, and bones.
Brain function: Copper is involved in the development and functioning of the central nervous system. It plays a role in the production of neurotransmitters, such as dopamine and norepinephrine, which are important for mood regulation and cognitive function.
Immune system support: Copper is necessary for the proper functioning of the immune system. It helps in the production of white blood cells, which are responsible for fighting off infections and foreign invaders.
Natural occurrence: Copper is widely distributed in nature and is found in various foods, including organ meats, shellfish, nuts, seeds, and whole grains. It can also be obtained through drinking water from copper pipes or cookware.
While copper is essential for the human body, excessive intake can be harmful. High levels of copper can lead to copper toxicity, which can cause symptoms such as nausea, vomiting, abdominal pain, and liver damage. It is important to maintain a balanced intake of copper through a varied and nutritious diet.
Foods sources of Copper:
Organ meats: Liver, especially beef liver, is one of the richest sources of copper, with about 12 mg per 100 grams. Other organ meats like kidney and heart also contain significant amounts of copper.

Shellfish: Oysters and mussels are good sources of copper, with around 6-7 mg per 100 grams. Other shellfish like crab and lobster also contain smaller amounts of copper.

Nuts and seeds: Cashews, almonds, and sesame seeds are all good sources of copper. They typically contain around 1-2 mg per 100 grams.

Legumes: Lentils, chickpeas, and soybeans are all good sources of copper. They typically contain around 1-2 mg per 100 grams.

Dark chocolate: Dark chocolate with a high cocoa content is a good source of copper. It typically contains around 1-2 mg per 100 grams.

Whole grains: Whole grains like oats, quinoa, and barley contain copper, although the amounts are relatively small compared to other sources. They typically provide around 0.5-1 mg per 100 grams.

Fruits: Some fruits like avocados, bananas, and prunes contain small amounts of copper. However, the copper content in fruits is generally lower compared to other sources.

The copper content can vary depending on factors such as soil quality, processing methods, and cooking techniques.

Selenium

Selenium is a chemical element that is classified as a nonmetal and belongs to the group 16 (chalcogens) of the periodic table. It has the atomic number 34 and the symbol Se. Selenium is a trace element that is essential for the human body in small quantities. It is found in soil, water, and certain foods. Selenium plays a crucial role in various biological processes, including antioxidant defense, thyroid hormone metabolism, and immune function. It is also known for its potential health benefits, such as reducing the risk of certain types of cancer and supporting reproductive health. However, excessive intake of selenium can be toxic, so it is important to maintain a balanced intake.

The selenium content can vary depending on factors such as soil quality, processing methods, and cooking techniques.

Foods sources of Selenium:

Brazil nuts: Brazil nuts are the richest source of selenium, with about 1917 mcg per 100 grams. Just a few Brazil nuts can provide your daily recommended intake of selenium.

Seafood: Fish and shellfish are good sources of selenium. Tuna, halibut, sardines, and shrimp all contain significant amounts of selenium.

Meat: Beef, lamb, and pork are good sources of selenium, with around 20-30 mcg per 100 grams. Chicken and turkey also contain smaller amounts of selenium.
Eggs: Eggs are a good source of selenium, with around 15-20 mcg per 100 grams.
Whole grains: Whole grains like wheat, rice, and oats contain selenium, although the amounts are relatively small compared to other sources. They typically provide around 10-20 mcg per 100 grams.
Legumes: Legumes like lentils, chickpeas, and beans contain selenium. They typically provide around 5-10 mcg per 100 grams.
Dairy products: Milk and cheese contain small amounts of selenium, with around 5-10 mcg per 100 grams. Yogurt and other dairy products also contain smaller amounts of selenium.
Vegetables: Some vegetables like mushrooms, spinach, and broccoli contain small amounts of selenium. However, the selenium content in vegetables is generally lower compared to other sources.

Iodine

Iodine is a chemical element that belongs to the group 17 (halogens) of the periodic table. It has the atomic number 53 and the symbol I. It is primarily found in seawater, rocks, and soils. Two-thirds of the body's iodine is in the thyroid gland.
Iodine is an essential micronutrient for the human body, meaning that it is required in small amounts to maintain good health. It is a crucial component of thyroid hormones, which regulate the body's metabolism and play a role in growth, development, and maintaining body temperature. Adequate iodine intake is especially important during pregnancy for fetal brain development. An undersupply of this mineral can result in slow mental reaction, weight gain, and lack of energy.
Iodine deficiency can lead to various health problems, including goiter (enlargement of the thyroid gland), hypothyroidism (underactive thyroid), and impaired cognitive function. To prevent iodine deficiency, iodized salt is commonly used to ensure sufficient iodine intake in many parts of the world. The iodine content in foods can vary depending on factors such as soil quality, farming practices, and processing methods. Excessive intake of iodine can also have adverse effects on health, so it is important to maintain a balanced intake within recommended limits.
Foods sources of Iodine:
Seafood: Seaweed and seafood are the richest sources of iodine. Seaweed, such as kelp and nori, can contain extremely high levels of iodine. Fish like cod, tuna, and shrimp also contain significant amounts of iodine.

Dairy products: Milk, yogurt, and cheese are good sources of iodine. Dairy products from cows that have been fed iodine-rich feed can have higher iodine content.
Eggs: Eggs are a good source of iodine, with around 20-30 mcg per egg.
Iodized salt: Iodized salt is a common source of iodine. It is regular table salt that has been fortified with iodine. However, excessive salt intake can have negative health effects, so it is best to consume iodized salt in moderation.
Seaweed and sea vegetables: Seaweed, such as kelp, nori, and wakame, are excellent sources of iodine. They can be consumed in various forms, such as in sushi, salads, or as a seasoning.
Some fruits and vegetables: Fruits and vegetables are not typically rich sources of iodine. Certain fruits and vegetables can contain decent amounts if they are grown in iodine-rich soil. Examples include strawberries, cranberries, spinach, green beans, navy beans, and potatoes (especially the skin).

Manganese

Manganese is a chemical element that belongs to the group 7 (transition metals) of the periodic table. It has the atomic number 25 and the symbol Mn. Manganese is a gray-white metal and is commonly found in minerals such as pyrolusite, rhodochrosite, and braunite.
Manganese plays a vital role in various biological processes in the human body.
It is an essential trace element that is involved in the metabolism of carbohydrates, cholesterol, and amino acids. Manganese also acts as a cofactor for several enzymes involved in antioxidant defense, bone formation, and the synthesis of certain hormones.
While manganese deficiency is rare, a severe deficiency can lead to impaired growth, skeletal abnormalities, and problems with glucose metabolism.
Excessive intake of manganese can be harmful to health. Prolonged exposure to high levels of manganese, such as through inhalation of manganese dust or fumes in certain occupational settings, can lead to a condition called manganism. Symptoms of manganism can include movement disorders, tremors, and cognitive impairments.
It is important to maintain a balanced intake of manganese through a well-rounded diet and to avoid excessive exposure to high levels of manganese.
Foods sources of Manganese:
Nuts and seeds: Nuts and seeds are excellent sources of manganese. Pumpkin seeds, flaxseeds, sesame seeds, and almonds are particularly high in manganese.

Whole grains: Whole grains like oats, brown rice, quinoa, and whole wheat are good sources of manganese. They typically contain higher levels of manganese compared to refined grains.

Legumes: Legumes like chickpeas, lentils, and black beans are good sources of manganese. They are also rich in other nutrients like fiber and protein.

Leafy green vegetables: Leafy greens like spinach, kale, and Swiss chard contain manganese. These vegetables are also packed with other vitamins and minerals.

Tea: Certain types of tea, such as black tea and green tea, contain manganese. However, the manganese content can vary depending on the brewing method and brand.

Pineapple: Pineapple is a fruit that contains manganese. It is also a good source of vitamin C and other antioxidants.

Seafood: Some types of seafood, such as mussels and clams, contain manganese. They are also rich in other minerals like zinc and iron.

Spices: Certain spices, such as cloves, cinnamon, and turmeric, contain manganese. The manganese content can vary depending on factors such as soil quality, farming practices, and processing methods.

Molybdenum

Molybdenum is a trace mineral that is essential for various biological processes in the body. It is found in small amounts in food and is required in very small quantities for normal growth and development. Molybdenum plays a crucial role in the metabolism of amino acids, which are the building blocks of proteins. It also acts as a cofactor for several enzymes involved in important chemical reactions in the body. Molybdenum is involved in the metabolism of certain drugs and toxins, as well as the detoxification of sulfites. Although molybdenum deficiency is rare, it can lead to symptoms such as fatigue, rapid heart rate, and increased susceptibility to infections.

The exact molybdenum content in foods can vary depending on factors such as soil quality and farming practices.

Foods sources of Molybdenum:

Legumes: Legumes like lentils, peas, and beans are excellent sources of molybdenum. They are also high in protein, fiber, and other minerals.

Whole Grains: Whole grains like oats, brown rice, and quinoa contain molybdenum. They are also high in fiber, vitamins, and minerals.

Nuts and Seeds: Nuts and seeds such as almonds, walnuts, sunflower seeds, and sesame seeds are good sources of molybdenum. They are also rich in healthy fats and provide other essential nutrients.

Leafy Green Vegetables: Vegetables like spinach, kale, and broccoli are not only rich in molybdenum but also provide a wide range of other nutrients like vitamins A, C, and K, as well as folate.

Organ Meats: Organ meats like liver and kidney are good sources of molybdenum. However, they are also high in cholesterol, so they should be consumed in moderation.

Dairy Products: Dairy products like milk and cheese contain molybdenum. They are also rich in calcium, protein, and other essential minerals.

Nickel and Vanadium

Nickel and vanadium, although present in minuscule quantities within the human body, play roles that are not as clearly defined as those of other trace minerals. Although they are classified as trace minerals, their consumption in excess can lead to harmful effects, given the incredibly small quantities required by the body.

These elements are found in a modest variety of foods in minor amounts. The dietary intake of most individuals typically provides sufficient quantities of these minerals, negating the need for supplementary intake, which could potentially result in harmful effects if administered in large doses.

Nickel

Nickel (Ni): Nickel is thought to be involved in the body's metabolic processes. It may play a role in the production of red blood cells and helps the body absorb and utilize various nutrients. However, excessive nickel can be toxic, so it's important to maintain a balance. Foods that contain nickel include nuts and seeds, whole grains, dried fruits, chocolate, and certain types of fish and shellfish. It can also be found in some drinking water and in certain cooking utensils.

Vanadium

Vanadium (V): Vanadium is believed to play a role in bone development and in metabolism, particularly in the regulation of blood sugar levels. Some research suggests it may mimic the actions of insulin. However, the body's requirement for vanadium is not well established and excessive amounts can be harmful. You can find vanadium in mushrooms, shellfish, black pepper, parsley, dill weed, beer, wine, grain and grain products, and artificially sweetened drinks.

Good Nutrition to Reduce Stress

Several vitamins and minerals are known to help reduce stress levels. These include:
B Vitamins: The B-vitamin family, including B1 (thiamine), B2 (riboflavin), B3 (niacin), B5 (pantothenic acid), B6 (pyridoxine), B7 (biotin), B9 (folate or folic acid), and B12 (cobalamins), play crucial roles in brain health and the production of stress-regulating hormones. They can be found in whole grains, meat, eggs, legumes, seeds, and nuts.
Vitamin C: This vitamin is essential for the production of stress hormones in the adrenal glands. It's found in citrus fruits, strawberries, bell peppers, and broccoli.
Magnesium: Known as the "relaxation mineral," magnesium plays a role in functions including nerve transmission and muscle relaxation. It's found in foods like leafy green vegetables, nuts, seeds, legumes, and whole grains.
Zinc: Zinc is crucial for the immune system and brain health, both of which can be affected by stress. It's found in meats, shellfish, legumes, nuts, and seeds.
Omega-3 Fatty Acids: While not a vitamin or mineral, these fatty acids are worth mentioning as they can help regulate mood and maintain brain health. They are found in fatty fish, walnuts, flaxseeds, and chia seeds.
Vitamin D: Often known as the "sunshine vitamin," Vitamin D can help regulate mood and reduce feelings of anxiety and depression. It's found in fatty fish, egg yolks, and fortified dairy products, but can also be synthesized by the body in response to sunlight.
Ways good nutrition helps to manage and reduce stress:
Balanced Blood Sugar: Consuming balanced meals and snacks with proteins, fiber, and healthy fats throughout the day can help maintain stable blood sugar levels, reducing swings in energy and mood.
Stress-Busting Nutrients: Certain nutrients like Vitamin B complex, Vitamin C, magnesium, and omega-3 fatty acids are known for their role in supporting the body's physical response to stress.
Gut Health: The gut and brain are closely linked. Consuming probiotic-rich foods like yogurt, kefir, and fermented foods can help maintain a healthy gut, which may influence mood and stress levels.
Reduced Caffeine and Sugar: Both can cause energy spikes and crashes throughout the day, and may increase feelings of anxiety and stress.
Hydration: Even mild dehydration can affect mood and energy levels. Drinking sufficient water throughout the day can help maintain hydration status and potentially reduce stress.
Mindful Eating: Paying attention to what and when you eat can help create a healthier relationship with food, reduce stress-related eating, and lead to better nutritional choices overall.

Conclusion: The Symphony of Nutrients

Nutrition and Health: A Lifelong Partnership

The journey through the world of vitamins and minerals culminates in a profound understanding of their vital role in human health. These micronutrients, though required in relatively small amounts, are essential for the intricate biochemical processes that sustain life. Proper nutrition, a cornerstone of well-being, hinges on the delicate balance and synergy of these nutrients, working in concert with macronutrients like proteins, carbohydrates, and fats.

Optimal nutrition signifies a state where all essential nutrients are supplied and utilized in harmonious balance, fueling the body's myriad functions and maintaining optimal health and well-being. This intricate interplay of nutrients orchestrates a symphony of biological processes, from energy production and cellular repair to immune function and cognitive performance. Let's recap the key players in this nutritional orchestra:

Macronutrients: The Energy Providers: Proteins, carbohydrates, and fats are the primary sources of energy, providing the fuel necessary for body heat, physical activity, and cellular function. Their energy potential is measured in calories, representing the amount of chemical energy released as heat during metabolism. Proteins, composed of amino acids, are the building blocks of tissues, enzymes, and hormones. Carbohydrates, the body's preferred energy source, are broken down into glucose to fuel cellular processes. Fats, essential for hormone production, cell membrane structure, and nutrient absorption, also provide a concentrated source of energy.

Micronutrients: The Regulators and Catalysts: Vitamins and minerals, though needed in smaller quantities, are indispensable for countless biochemical reactions. Vitamins, organic compounds, act as coenzymes, facilitating metabolic processes. Minerals, inorganic substances, play structural roles and participate in various cellular functions. These micronutrients work synergistically, orchestrating a complex network of biological activities that support optimal health.

The Foundation of a Healthy Life

Good nutrition is the bedrock of a healthy life, impacting every aspect of our physical and mental well-being. Its influence extends to:

Organ Development and Function: Adequate nutrition provides the building blocks and regulatory factors necessary for the healthy development and function of all organs.
Growth and Reproduction: From infancy to adulthood, proper nutrition supports growth, development, and reproductive health.
Immunity and Disease Resistance: A well-nourished body has a stronger immune system, better equipped to fight off infections and diseases.
Tissue Repair and Recovery: Nutrients are essential for repairing damaged tissues and recovering from injuries.

The Power of Synergy: Nutrition and Exercise

While proper nutrition provides the foundation for a healthy body, physical activity adds another vital dimension. Exercise complements good nutrition by:

Enhancing Organ Function: Regular exercise strengthens the cardiovascular system, improves lung capacity, and boosts metabolic function.
Maintaining Musculoskeletal Health: Exercise builds strong muscles and bones, promoting mobility and preventing age-related decline.
Improving Mental Well-being: Physical activity releases endorphins, natural mood boosters that reduce stress and improve mental clarity.

The synergy between nutrition and exercise creates a powerful force for optimal health, enhancing physical and mental well-being throughout the lifespan.

The Wisdom of Whole Foods

The benefits of vitamins and minerals are best achieved through a balanced diet that emphasizes whole, unprocessed foods. Fruits, vegetables, whole grains, lean proteins, and healthy fats provide a rich array of essential nutrients in their natural forms. These foods offer a synergistic blend of vitamins, minerals, fiber, and phytonutrients that work together to promote optimal health.

Supplements: A Complementary Role

While supplements can be helpful in addressing specific nutrient deficiencies or supporting particular health needs, they should not be considered a replacement for a healthy diet. Whole foods offer a complex matrix of nutrients that work synergistically, providing benefits that isolated supplements cannot replicate. Consult with a healthcare professional or registered dietitian before taking any supplements to determine their appropriateness and ensure safe and effective usage.

A Lifelong Commitment

Building healthy eating habits is a lifelong journey, not a destination. It requires conscious choices, mindful awareness, and a commitment to nourishing your body with the nutrients it needs to thrive. Embrace the abundance of nutritious and delicious foods available, experiment with new recipes, and savor the pleasures of healthy eating. By making informed choices and prioritizing nutrition, you invest in your present and future health, laying the foundation for a vibrant, energetic, and fulfilling life.

Beyond the Plate: A Holistic Approach

While this book has focused on the essential roles of vitamins and minerals, it's important to remember that nutrition is just one piece of the wellness puzzle. Other lifestyle factors, such as adequate sleep, stress management, regular physical activity, and maintaining positive social connections, also play crucial roles in overall health and well-being. By embracing a holistic approach that integrates these various elements, you can cultivate a vibrant and balanced life, maximizing your potential for health, happiness, and longevity. The journey towards optimal well-being is a lifelong adventure, and the knowledge you've gained about vitamins and minerals provides a strong foundation for navigating this path with confidence and success. May you continue to explore the fascinating world of nutrition and embrace the power of healthy living.

"The doctor of the future will no longer treat the human frame with drugs, but rather will cure and prevent disease with nutrition."
Thomas Edison